PELVIC PAIN

Lea Wilson

PELVIC PAIN

An American Surgeon
Liberates Himself

— *2014* —

Originated in United States of America by
Lea Wilson of MINDFUL LIFE SKILLS LLC.
Email: leawilson1342@yahoo.com.
Website: pelvicpain-cpps.com

Cover design by Kit Foster
Book design by Maureen Cutajar, www.gopublished.com

The material in this book is for information only. It may not be construed as medical advice or instruction. This book is not intended as a substitute for the medical advice of physicians. The reader should regularly consult a physician in matters relating to his/her health and particularly with respect to any symptoms that may require diagnosis or medical attention. This nonfiction book has been compiled from the author's own personal experiences and reading of multiple existing public references and published scientific studies. The story shared is a recollection to the best of the author's knowledge. The author does not guarantee the accuracy of the source materials or the personal conclusions drawn and disclaims liability for the accuracy of the information.

Ebook ISBN: 978-0-9960503-1-9
Print ISBN: 978-1-4995569-6-4

Library of Congress Catalog Number: 2014909175
Wilson, Lea, 1953 -
      Pelvic Pain: An American surgeon liberates himself / Lea Wilson.
      p. cm.
      ISBN 978-1-4995569-6-4 (pbk)
      Includes bibliographical references.

1. Pelvic pain. 2. Pelvic pain --Treatment. 3. Pelvis --Diseases --Treatment. 4. Pelvis --Physiopathology. 5. Chronic pain --Treatment. 6. Chronic pain --Alternative treatment. 7. Mindfulness-based cognitive therapy. 8. Meditation --Therapeutic use. I. Title.

Createspace Independent Publishing Platform
North Charleston, SC

*To my husband, for encouraging
me to follow my interests.*

[WISDOM]

"In the field of observation, chance favours only the prepared mind."

—Louis Pasteur

"This is your 35th attempt to elicit an emotional response from me."

—Young Spock

"Conscious experience not only requires an experiencer who has *learned* about the geography of its own representations, but it also requires experiencers who *care* about their experiences."

—Axel Cleeremans

"The important thing is they're doing a very new thing in a concerted way. And their brain says, hey, if we're going to be doing this thing in the environment over and over and over, I'm going to build tissue to do that so that we can do it easier and more efficiently. So if you're going to be creative, pick one thing, get a lot of experience in that one thing, and do it over and over and over."

—Rex Jung

[CONTENTS]

Introduction

A FEW YEARS AGO, I was watching as my husband's pelvic pain worsened in frequency and intensity. He could not take the long walks on the beach that were supposed to become one of the highlights of our retirement. He was okay during surgery but could not turn away from the operating room table without almost doubling over in pain. He was beginning to have a haggard look and a gray color in his face, adding ten years to his appearance. I have pictures from this time to remind us.

I was scared. Our future was being threatened, but the scariest part was that *his* future was being threatened. The years of delayed gratification, the years of hard work, and the years of sacrifice! How could this be happening to him?

This low point came after almost three years of following treatment protocols (diagnostic testing, drugs, physical therapy, National Center for Complementary and Alternative Medicine recommendations, dietary restrictions) currently outlined in world standards of care for the poorly understood *male chronic pelvic pain syndrome*. This low point just happened to coincide with a time in my life when I was avidly reading about three things – neuroplasticity, functional movement, and creativity.

As it turns out, this information formed the foundation of the plans for how my husband would work with his *body* and his *mind* in an effort to liberate himself. Success came in a much shorter time frame than we imagined.

This book is a telling of the work and practice of less than a year (June to November) that was successful.

This book does not represent medical advice.

[1]

Understanding Male Pelvic Pain

To be clear, the type of pain that this book reports about is specific to a male, non-specific in external or internal initiation, difficult to localize, and elusive in obvious pathology.

CHRONIC PELVIC PAIN: What It Is

The many symptoms that accompany *chronic pelvic pain* are associated with various diagnoses: urological (chronic prostatitis, interstitial cystitis, urgency and frequency syndrome, painful bladder syndrome) and non-urological (cancer, stones, infections, and other potentially life-threatening conditions).

This complex problem is recognized to have nociceptive, visceral and neuropathic components, and is a diagnostic challenge to all health care providers. "Patients suffer considerable morbidity throughout their lives resulting in a significant decrease in quality of life for both the patient and his/her partner due to the physical and physiological impact…Studies involving a medical diagnosis suggest CP/CPPS (Chronic Prostatitis/Chronic Pelvic Pain Syndrome) affects as many as 9% of men while the prevalence of self-reported prostatitis-like symptoms has been estimated to be as high at 16%." Ref: Urologic Chronic Pelvic Pain Syndrome (UCPPS) Research (R01). National Institutes of Health Web site. http://grants.nih.gov/grants/guide/rfa-files/RFA-DK-12-025.html. Published November 30, 2012. Accessed September 1, 2013.

There are currently no universally effective therapies available, so the medical practitioner ends up managing the symptoms of the problem with a specific emphasis on the *management of pain.*

I decided that *liberation from pain* was a better goal.

MY READING LISTS

I read a lot of material related to the *mind and brain* mostly because I like knowing about a lot of things. My reading focused on:

> *neuro-plasticity, brain training, effects of mental training, psychophysiological assessments and biofeedback based interventions, self-monitoring, self-referential processing, cognitive monitoring, self-regulation, emotional intelligence, attention, attentional processing, working memory, executive function, cognitive behavioral therapy, relaxation response, thought suppression, regulation of urges, focusing, negativity bias, mirror neurons, self-control, willpower, acceptance and commitment therapy, mindsight, learned helplessness, fear conditioning, systematic mental training using motor imagery, process-specific learning, cognitive-control skills, cortical engagement, interoception, neuroticism, ironic process theory*

I was also exploring my interest in *aging and physical fitness*. I read about:

> *anatomy for fitness and wellness, biomechanics of resistance training, biomechanical precepts of posture, functional movement assessment, postural assessment, standardization of biomechanical alignment in yoga postures*

About this time, I was listening to podcasts about *learning, intelligence and creativity* because my fifty-year-old brother had two girls under the age of four years. I wanted to remind myself about what I knew about kids and review what had been learned since the last time I needed to know about "how not to mess with their heads." Some of the things discussed on the programs I listened to had me reading more about:

> *creativity, transient hypo-frontality, sleep, human skill set as more than just IQ, the nature of insight, "Aha!" moments, sleep-related insight, unlearning, cognitive and non-cognitive learning, non-conscious self-regulation, explicit, tacit and implicit memory*

With the *new incentive (my husband's pelvic pain)*, I began to read through a mountain of medical and scientific publications about:

> *chronic pelvic pain, pelvic floor problems, myofascia, myofascial slings, trigger point issues, sensory gating, diastasis, non-relaxing pelvic floor, levator ani syndrome,*

breath mechanics, paradoxical relaxation, attentional bi-as, priming, over-applied core stability training, dietary implications, pain-related emotions, brain maps, cognitive modulation of pain

I expanded my interests in *biomechanics* to include:

postural causes of pain, regional interdependence, breath accessory muscles, extensor coxae brevis and pelvic tilt, lower extremity consequences of core dysfunction, normal human locomotion

CONCLUSIONS ABOUT NORMAL BRAIN ACTIVITIES

Eventually, I had an image of a brain that is capable of practicing something (in this case pelvic pain) so often and so thoroughly that *the practice stimulates the brain to build neurologic connections both within and throughout the body that allow it to do the pain effortlessly and more efficiently*. The brain apparently ignores some information, amplifies other information, and generates or imagines spontaneous information specific to the practice.

These *normal brain activities* are a BONUS if you want to improve your golf game or to play wicked guitar, but they are devastating if the object of the brain's practice is pelvic pain. The brain can get very good at doing pelvic pain!

CONCLUSIONS ABOUT WHAT NEEDED TO BE DONE

1. This is very important to understand. It is not our fault that our brain is designed this way. Once we recognize our brain design though, it is our responsibility and choice to work with it.

2. We must admit that we don't know everything we need to know, and that's okay. Generally speaking, people who don't "leave their door open" to new information, rarely make great, new discoveries.

3. We come with a brain and body. That brain and body have practiced the "NO pelvic pain" longer than they have practiced pelvic pain, and that information is still stored in our long-term memories. You can't unlearn "NO pelvic pain" – it's stored in there somewhere!

4. The brain is plastic – its structure and function change in response to experience – even during sleep! And apparently, the changes occur in response to affective as well as sensorimotor experience, and in response to mental practice as well as physical practice.

5. Recent science is in agreement that the ability to redirect our attention leads to some physical, mental, and emotional trait changes. These changes can include the ability of our brain to regulate with flexibility not just emotions but also **autonomic functions** (This is BIG!), not just in the everyday conscious state but also in the subconscious states where the brain is a **creative, problem-solving organ**, cultivating solutions for use in our ordinary conscious state. Our creative brain is designed to assimilate new and old information into solutions. We need to provide lots of information and

     lots of opportunity for the brain to initiate the desired action and to avoid or correct errors.

6.   Attentional skills are trainable.

7.   Insight into the pain problem is insufficient to change lives. Action is required. There are no shortcuts here. Sustained effort is required.

8.   The action needed includes training cognitive functions for both our conscious state and the states that we are not conscious of, training many systems at the same time and training using a challenging variety in the exercises.

9.   The necessary action also includes giving the brain and body more recent experiences to provide a **distraction or redirection** from the "pain business as usual" processes, to provide a **reframing** of current experience, to initiate and encourage a creative solution and to initiate and encourage a remembrance of past pain-free processes.

CONVINCING MY HUSBAND

After my husband had been free from his pelvic pain for a year, I was describing what had happened to a friend who is also a family medical doctor. He said that he didn't think that most of his patients would do what my husband did.

Why not? Because it involved the individual patient "doing" something for himself, "self-directed"? Because we have been trained as patients to look for "treatment"?

Even when people do seek treatment, compliance with recommendations is amazingly poor.

"Adherence to long-term therapy for chronic illnesses in developed countries averages 50%." Ref: Sabate´ E. 2003. *Adherence to Long-Term Therapies: Evidence for Action*. Geneva: World Health Organ.

"Generally speaking, it was estimated that the compliance rate of long-term medication therapies was between 40% and 50%. The rate of compliance for short-term therapy was much higher at between 70% and 80%, while the compliance with lifestyle changes was the lowest at 20%–30%." Ref: Jin J, Sklar GE, Min Sen Oh V, Chuen Li S. Factors affecting therapeutic compliance: A review from the patient's perspective. Ther Clin Risk Manag. 2008; 4(1): 269–286.

My friend knows these numbers. Given these statistics, he may be right about most people.

I told him that I thought that when a person experienced the amount and intensity of pain that my husband was experiencing, that person gets some self-direction. That person will try just about anything, especially if it was evidence-based and made sense.

Since my conclusions were evidence-based and made sense, it was not hard to convince my husband to try this self-directed plan. He was highly motivated!

THE PLAN

I outlined these goals for the plan:

1. Train his *attention* skills and improve his skills of *self-monitoring* and *redirection* using a Mental Practice Sequence.

2. Using his new skills, work daily in specific ways with *thought and emotion* that are part of the pelvic pain complex.

3. Using his new skills, work daily in specific ways with *physical posture, position and movement* that are part of the pelvic pain complex.

4. No change in other variables.
   Continue with diet restrictions that he had been adhering to for greater than two years. Also by this time, *he was not using any medication or other therapies.*

The plan was simple: Give his brain some new experiences, some distraction, some redirection, some reframing and *get out of its way!* The brain is a creative, problem-solving organ.

JUNE TO NOVEMBER

He started without delay. He got instructions for the basic drill for attention training in June and began his practice. For the next several months, I gave him suggestions and reminders almost daily for what he might choose to do on that day. By the time we went on vacation in November, he was pain free. (He still had urinary hesitancy. See Chapter 5 for how that was resolved.)

NOTE: Different approaches in medical treatment.

There is a point that I would like to make when talking about the use of different approaches in medical treatment. I explain it like this.

My husband finished his surgical residency training in 1986.

Question: Given the exponential advances in the diagnosis and treatment of breast cancer, if my husband still cared for patients the way he was trained in the late 80s, could he be "malpracticing"?

Now consider this: Research in many fields, many disciplines, is discovering how the brain works – a lot of it counterintuitive to the way we have thought about decision-making, willpower and learned behaviors.

Question: Why is it that we do not look at the *advances in medical knowledge of brain function* in the same way as advances in medical knowledge of breast cancer? If physicians and therapists ignore the advances in this area of science and the implications for diagnosis and treatment, are they "malpracticing"?

NOTE: The *training model* for *both* mental practice and physical practice.

My description to my husband of *how to train* mimics other common forms of *informal, self-directed training models*. I specified a *sequence of drills and exercises* that would take him through the same *stages* he would go through if he wanted to acquire the skill of playing guitar or golf – figuring out the basic skill, understanding and refining the basic skill and performing the basic skill automatically.

It is easy to understand that if you want to play golf or guitar really well that you must practice, practice some more, and practice beyond what it takes to learn the skill. The basic drills of the physical practice are repetitive. They require some conscious cognition. They require cognition in the subconscious that you would not be aware of. The repetitive practice changes and reorganizes tissue and connections in your body and your brain to make the basic aspects of your golf game or guitar playing more automatic and reflexive.

The exercises to train attention are no different. By repetitive drills of brain exercises (*the mental practice*), you change and reorganize connections in your brain to make basic aspects of your attention skills more automatic and reflexive.

What may be different about these training exercises in this instance is *the conscious intention to target different functional areas* of the brain.

Remember the premise: different experiential input to affective, as well as sensorimotor areas, using *mental* practice, as well as *physical* practice, is what will encourage the brain to be creative in solving the problem.

NOTE: Areas providing opportunity for new experiences and redirection.

1. *Thought, emotion, and sensations that are part of the pelvic pain complex.*

   Thoughts are volunteered by my husband's brain into his field of awareness. For example, his brain doesn't ask for his conscious *permission* or his conscious *effort* to generate some thoughts. Normally, he is *not* impressed about how spontaneous these thoughts are. The brain does this naturally. In a typical brain's day, thoughts come…thoughts come…thoughts come. Sometimes emotion and sensations come with the thoughts.

2. *Physical posture, position and movement that are part of
    the pelvic pain complex.*

    Posture, position and movements of his body are not
    normally noticed. For example, he stands, walks, sits,
    and so on. In his autopilot mode, he is *not* thinking
    about how his body does these things.

Training Attention Using a Mental Practice Sequence

At this point, you may really want to skip to the physical action part of this book. Please do not because the attention skill happens to be absolutely crucial in both the physical and the mental aspects of this liberation work. It is also one of the most important skills to have as a human, a necessity. It is a skill that most people are clueless about, and a skill that is not normally taught to us as children. Humans need to understand and study attention as a skill that can be trained and attention training as an activity that can produce changes in brain structure, neural circuits, and behavior.

UNDERSTANDING WHAT ATTENTION IS

Have you ever said that your "attention" was wandering? How did you know? How do you know that you have an "attention"? What is this thing you call your "attention"? Do you keep track of your "attention"? Why should you know where it is? If you wanted to understand more about your "attention" and how to train to be more skillful with it, what would you do? How long should it take to train your "attention"?

"Most of the time, we seem to be 'bombarded' by numerous stimuli coming in through all of our senses at the same time. Despite this, we usually have no difficulty in focusing attention on one stimulus while ignoring others, and this suggests that we have an exceptional ability to filter out unwanted stimuli. Further, because this act seems effortless and because we are unaware of how we do it, we have the illusion that it is a simple and straightforward process." Ref: Eamon Fulcher. *Cognitive Psychology*. Exeter, UK: Learning Matters Ltd; 2003.

Posner and Peterson identified three major cognitive functions for the attention system: orienting to sensory events, detecting signals for focused processing, and maintaining a vigilant or alert state. Ref: Posner MI, Peterson SE. The attention system of the human brain. Annu Rev Neurosci. 1990; 13: 25–42.

"…the ability to focus and sustain attention on an intended object requires skills involved in monitoring the focus of attention and detecting distraction, disengaging attention from the source of distraction, and (re)directing and engaging attention to the intended object." Ref: Lutz A, Slagter HA, Dunne J, Davidson RJ. Attention regulation and monitoring in meditation. Trends Cogn. Sci. 2008; 12: 163–169.

"Cognitive processes affecting attention can be developed and improved by training. The types of attentional skills that can be learned for specific sports include the ability to select the correct stimuli to attend to, the ability to shift attention, when appropriate, from one set of stimuli to another, and the ability to sustain attention. These skills are needed for success in most sports." Ref: The Oxford Dictionary of Sports Science & Medicine. 3rd ed. New York, NY: Oxford University Press; 2007.

"Although human experience is determined by the way people direct their attention, it is evident that they do not have complete control over such direction." Ref: McCallum CW. "Attention." *Encyclopaedia Britannica*. 2007. *Britannica Online*. Web. 29 Sept. 2013.

THE NECESSITY TO TRAIN ATTENTION SKILLS

Why did I believe that my husband should begin by training his attention? *Because he needed physical, mental, and emotional trait changes that come from the ability to redirect attention at key opportunities.*

The assumption was that, with improved attentional skills, he could *reflexively identify* the arising opportunities and then respond efficiently and effortlessly with *redirection*, interfering with the old ways of doing things. He could select how to work in a manner to increase the odds of getting "unstuck" from the pelvic pain.

As he was going about his day, it was critical for him to *reflexively identify* these windows of opportunity. The identification, selection, and redirection needed to be automatic. For this, he needed to almost "overlearn" the skill of attention, practicing to get really good at knowing where his attention was and really good at redirecting his attention to where he wanted it to be. This is where he had to begin.

My husband began with the mental practice.

INSTRUCTIONS FOR THE MENTAL PRACTICE SEQUENCE: The basic drill for training attention, self-monitoring, and redirection.

I present the instructions for the drill and practice in the four-part sequence that I suggested to my husband. With the attitude and intention of compassion, he first learned to monitor where his attention was, and then he strengthened the ability to put his attention where he wanted it. I provided suggestions for working with content and distraction that arose during his practice of the basic exercises. I kept it very simple.

1. To learn where his attention was:
In order to learn how to monitor where his attention was, I gave these instructions to keep his attention "focused" on one thing, his breath:

Sit in a comfortable position maintaining good anatomical posture.

Close your eyes.

Breathe normally through your nose – no breath manipulation.

Acknowledge your intention to access the abilities of the body and brain.

Acknowledge your intention to maintain a consistent focus and consistent observation.

Voluntarily allow the focus of your attention to be on the inhalational sensations of your breath (cooler air flowing into your nostrils, warming as it flows through the nasal cavity) and then the exhalational sensations of the warmed air.

Monitor, without force, to sustain your focus on the breath.

Recognize when your attention wanders, *note that it has wandered, choose to let go of whatever has engaged the attention without judgment, discourse, or rumination* and choose to bring your attention back to the breath sensations.

Monitor, without force, to sustain the feeling of being the observer.

Recognize when distracting thoughts are numerous and persistent. *Note the spontaneous flow and choose to let go without judgment, discourse, or rumination.* Choose to bring your attention back to the breath sensations.

I suggested that he practice this drill for fifteen to twenty minutes a day for two weeks before adding the second part.

> *Remember: It is not necessary to examine the content of the distractions at this time. There will be a time to work with content. This is not it. Whatever thought occurs is useful. (You can't work with your skill of disengaging attention from distracting thoughts if you have no thoughts!)*

2. To further strengthen his abilities and skills of attention.

To further strengthen the abilities and skills to identify where his attention was and to put his attention where he wanted it, I suggested that he "monitor" what was coming into his field of awareness but choose not to engage:

> Begin with your focus on your breath for a short while.

> Choose to decrease your focus on the breath.

> Choose to increase the sense of being an observer, focusing your attention on your field of awareness, your field of view that is being populated with information picked up by all of your sensory organs (smell, taste, touch, hearing, somatic, visceral, proprioceptions).

> As an observer, monitor your field of awareness and your mental activity or thoughts that arise within your field of awareness.

> Observe all of your mental activity in the field of awareness, much the same as you would look out a window of your house and observe the traffic that is going by, passes and continues down the street until it is out of sight, or as you imagine that you are standing on the command deck of a spaceship hurtling through deep space as you observe the space debris, shooting stars, and other spaceships that streak into your view and continue out of your sight into the darkness of space.

Recognize when your attention wanders, *note that it has wandered, choose to let go of whatever has engaged the attention without judgment, discourse, or rumination* and choose to bring your attention back to monitoring your field of awareness.

I suggested that he practice this drill fifteen to twenty minutes a day for two weeks until it felt familiar. Then add the third and fourth parts of the training.

> *Remember: This practice is for strengthening the attention "muscle" and does not work with content. The practice is with the "bare" display of what is occurring.*

> *The practice for working with content is addressed in the third and fourth parts.*

3. To work with the content of his thoughts in a general way.
To work with the content of his thoughts and input in a general way, I suggested that he note the content of the distracting thoughts (or whatever engaged his attention) in this manner:

Recognize when your attention wanders, and as the observer, note that it has wandered.

Choose to address what you are noting with simple comments or questions. *Do not answer your questions. Do not analyze or ruminate or elaborate.* Just silently ask the question or make the comment. Choose to limit yourself to several basic comments or questions:

- There is a thought.
- This is what the brain does. My brain contributes random thoughts.
- What it contributes may not be useful.
- The thought may have a story attached to it.
- I may need to examine this thought later.
- Where did that thought come from?
- Why does that thought keep appearing?

Choose to let go of whatever thought has engaged your attention without judgment, discourse, or rumination.

Choose to bring your attention back to observing your field of awareness.

4. To work with the content of his thoughts and emotions that are specifically about pelvic pain.

To work with the content of his thoughts and emotions that are specifically about pelvic pain, I suggested that he notice the content of the input in this manner, using specific refutations, redirections, or comments:

Recognize when your attention wanders, and as the observer, note that it has wandered.

Recognize when the thoughts are about pelvic pain issues.

Choose to address what you are noting with simple comments or questions. *Do not answer your questions. Do not analyze or ruminate or elaborate.* Just silently ask the question or make the comment. Use several basic comments or questions:

- There is a thought about my pelvic pain.
- This is what the brain does. My brain contributes thoughts.
- What it contributes may not be useful or accurate.
- I, like other feeling entities, wish to be happy and to be free from pain.

Choose to let go of whatever thought has engaged your attention.

Choose to bring your attention back to observing your field of awareness.

Remember: You do not need to address the content more specifically in this basic drill.

SUGGESTED SCHEDULE FOR THE MENTAL PRACTICE SEQUENCE

Remember: The Mental Practice Sequence is the basic drill for training attention, self-monitoring and redirection skills.

1. *Learn where your attention is. Practice this for two weeks.*
2. *Further strengthen your abilities and skills by monitoring what is coming into your "field of awareness" but choosing to not engage. Practice this for two weeks.*

From this time onward, when you sit down to practice, you may choose to spend a few minutes in the first part, then a few minutes in the second part before working with your content as per third and fourth parts.

3. *Choosing to engage with the content of your thoughts and input in a general way.*
4. *Choosing to engage with the content of your thoughts and emotions that are specifically about pelvic pain in a general way.*

From now on, you may find yourself switching between the parts of the drill during your practice. As you learn the changing nature of your field of awareness, you may return to the basic first part of practicing attention to breath. Other times, observing the content with or without engaging will be useful. It is your choice.

You will experience – just like learning any skill – that there is an ease, a familiarity, that comes with the consistency of frequent practice. How long will you use the basic skill practices? As with any basic strength, dexterity or flexibility skill, frequent practice aids in the maintenance of the skill. The initial month's work must be more like rehabilitation work – daily, with effort, referencing your instructions. After that, you will want a practice consistent with your goals.

PLEASE DO NOT MAKE THIS PRACTICE COMPLICATED!

I told my husband: Keep it simple. This *is* the basic drill for training attention skill.

I reminded him that this is the skill to be used every day to untangle the pelvic pain he had programed into his posture, movements, thoughts and emotions, so he needed to get good at it.

NOTE: Technical information.

It has not been shown that learning the *neuroscience of attention training* aids in getting the "action" done.

For those who are interested, more technical information including the *most recent research* is easily accessed online.

I am purposefully limiting the scope of this book to the simple practice that liberated my husband from his pain.

[3]

Working Daily in Specific Ways with Thoughts and Emotions

The day-to-day work on thought and emotional content entangled with pelvic pain builds on the basic drill. The basic drill work limits examination of content. The day-to-day work with content, all throughout the day, may include both limited examination (affecting what I call cognitive work happening in the brain without us being conscious of the work) and examination (what I call cognitive work happening in our conscious state). Both have a role to play in the untangling.

IDENTIFYING EVERYDAY OPPORTUNITIES FOR WORKING WITH THE THOUGHTS AND EMOTIONS THAT ARE PART OF THE PELVIC PAIN COMPLEX

Origins of the Content: All throughout his day, my husband could practice this new way of viewing and relating to his thoughts and feelings – that of being an observer acknowledging the content of his field of awareness in a structured way. He had access to his "self-awareness." He could differentiate and label the origins of the content.

1. The flow of information *produced by his brain in response to stimuli acting on sensory organs and tissue.* For example, sensations of sound, touch, etc.

2. The flow of mental events *spontaneously* (no effort on his part) *triggered and volunteered by his brain as it processed the sensations,* moving from the experience of the sensation to the experience of other mental chatter and stories (including thoughts and emotions).

3. The flow of mental events *coming from his conscious effort to control his brain and direct his thoughts* to either "problem solving or rumination" (not desirable as part of this practice) OR "identification, selection and redirection" (the desirable response).

These are opportunities to practice a different relationship to the origin of his content.

Themes of the Content: More and more, he skillfully recognized the thoughts and emotional content that were related to his pelvic pain. Several themes were common and bore resemblance to the three spirits that visited Scrooge in *A Christmas Carol.* Ref: Dickens C. *A Christmas Carol. In Prose. Being a Ghost Story of Christmas.* London: Chapman and Hall; 1843.

1. Recollections from the Past:
    "I have exhausted the available diagnostic and treatment modalities. Nothing helped. I have been having

pelvic pain for almost three years, and it is getting worse. My pelvic pain is affecting walking, sitting, sleeping, etc. All of this has been frustrating, maddening, saddening."

2. Ruminations about the Future:
    "My pelvic pain will only get worse. My retirement will suck because I will not be able to travel, enjoy beach activities – fishing, walking, surfing, kayaking. I will never be happy and free from pain again. Oh, no. I have to go again. Getting up from my desk may trigger my pain. Walking may trigger my pain."

3. Dealing with Present Time:
    "This pain is almost unbearable. Sitting quietly is not helping."

Yes! All three are specific opportunities to practice a different relationship to the themes using change, distraction, and redirection!

INSTRUCTIONS FOR PRACTICING EVERY DAY WITH THESE OPPORTUNITIES USING LIMITED EXAMINATION:

This is the daily work that I described to my husband as affecting cognitive activities by the brain that we are not conscious of.

He would do limited examination work in the conscious state, but the changes would take place "out of sight, out of mind," in his subconscious. Again I emphasized, this is evidence based and makes sense. Regardless of the origin or content of the thoughts, the instructions remained basically the same:

With the attitude and intention of compassion, acknowledge that the thought and emotional content observed is part of the contribution by the brain to the programming of his pelvic pain. Acknowledge that this observed programming might be illogical or faulty.

Acknowledge, as the observer, this "mental activity" about the pain.

Choose to remember that your brain contributes this "mental chatter" into your field of awareness.

Choose to address what you are noting with simple comments or questions. *Do not answer your questions. Do not analyze or ruminate or elaborate.* Just silently ask the question or make the comment. Use several of these basic comments or questions:

- There is a thought about my pelvic pain.
- This is what the brain does. My brain contributes thought.
- What it contributes may not be useful or accurate.
- The thought may have a story attached to it.
- I may need to examine this thought at a later time.

- Where did that thought come from?
- Why does that thought keep appearing?
- I, like other feeling entities, wish to be happy and to be free from pain.

Choose to let go of whatever thought has engaged your attention.

Choose to bring your attention back to what is happening in your day.

Note: There is no need to address the content more specifically.

As he practiced, my husband noted that the thoughts he observed would sometimes automatically elicit other content or events, some *intentionally generated with effort* (thinking, planning, evaluating, and interpreting) and some *not intentional* (mind wandering, daydreaming, ruminating). I reminded him the instructions remain the same – use limited examination.

At some point, he noted that there could be a different "felt" quality to some of the content, sometimes subtle and sometimes piercing. Would he call this anxiety? Again, I reminded him the instructions remain the same – use limited examination.

Sometimes, the thoughts and sensations coming into his field of awareness *was* the pelvic pain. With pelvic pain can come the *story* of the past (I've had this forever), the future (It will never get better), and the present (This hurts like hell! I don't think I can walk normally).

I reminded my husband that the brain could be wrong or not "totally right" in the situation – that it could be stuck in misinformation. The instructions for *dealing with the story* remain basically the same – choose to use *limited examination*.

> *Remember: The work here is about the story, not the "felt" sense of pain. Felt senses are addressed in Chapter 4.*

KEEP IT SIMPLE

My recommendation was to keep the everyday practice simple: **choose several comments that he could use in all situations** and practice them so that response to the thoughts would be *reflexive*. Use others as appropriate (sometimes it is obvious).

INSTRUCTIONS FOR PRACTICING WITH THESE OPPORTUNITIES USING EXAMINATION – COGNITIVE WORK IN THE CONSCIOUS STATE WITH PROFESSIONAL HELP

During the daily work outlined above, I told my husband to note if he found himself favoring comments similar to these:

- The thought may have a story attached to it.
- I may need to examine this thought at a later time.

With the attitude and intention of compassion, he would need to acknowledge that this recurring thought and emotional content that he was observing was part of the contribution by the brain to the programming of his pelvic pain. He must be aware that the *closer examination* of certain thought content can elicit in some people further *thought content and events that may potentially be harmful.*

In this situation, *professional help must be considered* to gain insight into how to work with these thoughts. This type of help was outside of my "scope of practice."

THE NECESSITY FOR PROFESSIONAL HELP

Stress, depression, and other psychological factors have been studied in relationship to chronic pelvic pain syndrome (CPPS), as well as chronic prostatitis (CP). In the results of one study, researchers found: "Men who reported having experienced sexual, physical, or emotional abuse had increased odds (1.7–3.3) for symptoms suggestive of CP/CPPS." Ref: Hu JC, Link CL, McNaughton-Collins M, Barry MJ, McKinlay JB. The association of abuse and symptoms suggestive of chronic prostatitis/chronic pelvic pain syndrome: results from the Boston Area Community Health survey. J Gen Intern Med. 2007; 22(11): 1532–7.

There is plenty of evidence that psychological histories should be taken seriously when considering what kind of work needs to be done when a person has pelvic pain. Many therapeutic modalities and cognitive-behavioral modalities used by psychotherapists would be appropriate in working with these issues.

It is true that many people never seek help in dealing with serious psychological issues or with personality disorders. Both can prevent progress in the liberation from pelvic pain. Self-help may be effective but may take far longer than using experienced psychological help. Not recognizing the need for help may doom the recovery or worse.

In the examination of the content of his thoughts and emotions, my husband did not identify content that he needed to "examine later," to purposefully work with in a conscious manner, at a later date. If he had identified areas that he delayed for examination, I would have encouraged him to seek professional help.

Choosing Professional Help

My husband was fortunate. If he had required assistance, we would have looked for therapists who described their practices with the following approaches:

> *CBT (cognitive behavioral therapy), DBT (dialectical behavioral therapy), ACT (acceptance and commitment therapy), EFT (emotionally focused therapy), focusing, SFBT (solution-focused brief therapy), MBCT (mindfulness based cognitive therapy), Motivational Interviewing, compassion-focused therapy, psychodynamic / psychoanalytic therapy, somatic/body therapies, and somatic experiencing.*

NOTE: Brain functioning.

Working on the past, present, and future is typical content for brain activity.

This is the brain functioning as it is designed and as it has been programmed. It delivers thoughts and emotions into the field of awareness. It generates this content using current sensory experience, and experience retrieved from short-term and long-term memory. (Memory encoded by the brain after it had received sensory information, interpreted and translated the information, associated it with other information, acted on it and then stored it.)

Some of the stored memory can also be "wired" to various body parts, so the memory has a "felt" quality – such as a feeling of great joy or satisfaction, a sick feeling in the stomach, a broken heart.

What is important to remember is that this brain system that we are using may have faults all along, in reception, translation, processing, storage, and retrieval.

What fires together, wires together!

NOTE: Cognitive activities by the brain that we are not conscious of.

We can be grateful that our brain is capable of this.

Could you imagine an alternative where everything that happened in our body had to be brought into our field of awareness where we would be conscious of the process and/or activity? It would be exhausting.

[4]

Working Daily in Specific Ways with Posture, Position, and Movement

The day-to-day work on postural and neuromuscular memories entangled with pelvic pain uses the improved attention skill to assist in identifying distraction and redirection opportunities throughout the day and in implementing the prescribed instructions.

ROLE OF POSTURE AND POSITION IN CHRONIC PAIN

There is a lot written by many health practitioners about the role of posture and biomechanics in all kinds of pain. In rehabilitation medicine, physical therapy, Rolfing, Alexander technique, massage therapy, and yoga as therapy, posture evaluation is a major part of an assessment.

It's hard to tell from the scientific literature just how important it is. Much research is devoted to the effects of postures and positions assumed at home, at work, and during sleep.

Some studies focus on positions that increase pressure on nerves and put muscles in shortened positions, so that other muscles get elongated. This results in other muscles being overused and reportedly leads to pain in some situations.

These muscle imbalances can happen anywhere in the body. This suggests posture and position could have a role in pelvic pain.

Adding to this puzzle is the fact that even if posture is as important as people want to believe, healthcare practitioners are not efficient in assessing it. Ref: Fedorak C, Ashworth N, Marshall J, Paull H. Reliability of the visual assessment of cervical and lumbar lordosis: how good are we? Spine. 2003; 28(16): 1857-9.

That said, my husband and I were not looking for specific postural "imbalances" that were causing pelvic pain. The goal of our assessment was to identify overall postural elements in various body positions that might be candidates for a small change, *a small redirection*. We did not need to be "good" at postural evaluation.

Most of my husband's symptoms were in anatomical structures located somewhere below the belly button and above the thighs, the pelvic area. This, along with the idea that unrelated structures and "wiring" in the region might be contributing to his experience of pelvic pain, suggested what needed to be done without being specific about the anatomy or his posture.

ELEMENTS TO EVALUATE: IDENTIFYING EVERYDAY OPPORTUNITIES FOR WORKING WITH PHYSICAL POSTURE, POSITIONS AND MOVEMENTS THAT ARE PART OF THE PELVIC PAIN COMPLEX

In describing this part of the plan to my husband, I reminded him of the premise that the variety of recent experiences in sensorimotor areas, using mental practice, as well as physical practice, is what will encourage the brain to be creative in solving his problem.

He is well aware of the anatomy of the area below the belly button and above the thighs. He understood how much of his movement during the day involved this area. He saw lots of potential for the introduction of new and different sensory experience into his posture, position, and movement.

We considered the following **elements to evaluate**:

- Posture, position, and changes in position
- Movements
- Sitting and sleeping ergonomics
- External physical stimuli
- Felt senses
- Thought content

Posture, position, and changes in position
Overall, postural elements that could appear to deviate from normal/neutral in different body positions: standing, sitting, squatting, lying, kneeling, and crouching.

- Specific postural elements in the pelvic area.
- Position changes made throughout the day – sitting

to standing, standing to sitting, standing to standing
forward bend, change in sleeping position.

Result: When we looked at my husband's posture, using information from Internet searches as a guide, we thought that he
did deviate from "normal" in ways typical of *old surgeons* (just
go to any meeting of surgeons, and you will see what I mean).
He had a slight drooping of his chest. Along with the chest sag,
his shoulders were rounding forward, his head and neck lean-
ing way forward with his shoulder blades spreading away and
up from the middle of his back. His shoulders were slightly
behind his hips (or pelvis shifted forward in space). We could
also see that he had a noticeable, almost exaggerated forward
tilt of his pelvis. These deviations from "normal" could appear
in all positions –standing, sitting, resting, sleeping, movement,
working, operating.

Movements
Movements made throughout a day – walking (human locomotion), walking up/down stairs, movements during work,
turning, standing up, and sitting down.

Results: We reviewed normal human locomotion and movements using references from the Internet and identified that,
with his shoulders slightly behind his hips, he had a stiffness in
his pelvis during the swing phase of walking, which seemed to
affect the flexing and lifting of his thighs. His feet led with toes
pointed so that his foot-strike ended more on his toes than his
heel. We also decided he should not try to remember military
posture.

Sitting and sleeping ergonomics
Posture during sitting or sleeping.

Results: We evaluated the basic ergonomics of every seat that he habitually used during his day – at home, in his car, at work – and of every bed that he sleeps in.

External physical stimuli
Other ways to introduce new experiences to his soft tissues using pressure and heat.

Results: We reviewed and borrowed techniques and tools from physical therapy, massage therapy, and myofascial therapy.

Felt senses
The concept of mental full-body scan or scan of specific areas of the body (systematic "inventory" of body areas, focusing on the body sensations) that may have linkages to his programmed pelvic pain.

Results: I reviewed philosophy and transcripts for body scan practices.

Thought content
Thought content specific to the body, body movement, and pelvic pain.

Results: We identified his common thought patterns specifically about body felt senses, body posture, body positions, and body movement during pain.

INSTRUCTIONS FOR WORKING WITH PHYSICAL POSTURES, POSITIONS AND MOVEMENTS THAT ARE PART OF THE PELVIC PAIN COMPLEX

The kinds of changes that could be made include:
- *correction and redirection*
- *introducing new experiences*
- *introducing more variety of experiences*

I gave these instructions:
- Keep it very simple with ***tiny changes***.
- Avoid exaggeration.
- Choose the attitude and intention of compassion.
- Choose to look for opportunities for practice throughout the day.

Posture, position, changes in position and movement:

Sometimes, during your day when you are sitting, standing, or lying down, choose to specifically *"take an inventory"* of your body. To feel your alignment, refer to what you understand as "neutral posture" for each part of your body. Then tune into your body, begin at your feet and move up your body with your examination – feet, ankle, calf, knee, thigh, hips, buttocks, pelvic area, abdomen, spine, chest, back, shoulders, upper arm, lower arm, hand, neck, face and head.

Choose to make tiny, conscious changes in what has been your default posture. Refer to the mountain pose of yoga postures: feet hip distance apart, equal external rotation of feet and legs, knees equally flexed and extended with no hyper-flexion, hip points level, lengthen your spine, ears over shoulders, shoulder blades toward the middle of the back and down slightly, a belly button awareness with a slight movement towards the spine.

Specifically choose to make a *tiny*, conscious change in your pelvic tilt, slightly decreasing the anterior tilt of your pelvis.

Sometimes, during your day when standing, see if you can feel the position of your pelvis. Choose to make a *tiny*, conscious change in your pelvic tilt, slightly decreasing the anterior tilt of your pelvis.

Sometimes, during your day when sitting, see if you can feel that you are on your "sitting bones." Choose to make a *tiny*, conscious change in your pelvic tilt, slightly decreasing the anterior tilt of your pelvis.

Sometimes, during your day, choose to specifically tune in to your movements. When you start to stand up, or you start to sit (in your chair at your desk, in the seat of the car, etc.) pause for a moment to "scan" your posture, choosing to specifically target the feeling of your pelvic position. Choose to make a *tiny*, conscious change in your pelvic tilt.

Remember: "Everything is a *squat*."

In the operating room, when you are finished with a surgical procedure, pause for a moment before leaving the operating table to "scan" your posture. Make *tiny*, conscious changes particularly in your pelvic tilt. Tune into the feeling of the lifting leg as it swings from the hip to take a turning step away from the table.

Sometimes, during your day, choose to specifically tune in to your walking motions, on flat surfaces or when climbing stairs. Choose, when you start to walk, to tune in to the feeling of lifting your leg using your hip flexor muscles, feeling your leg swing forward from your hip. Feel your heel touch the ground, and then the movement of your ankle as the sole of your foot and then the toes make the connection for push-off (heel-sole-toe). Feel the rotation (internal/external) of your leg (thigh, knee and feet should be same).

Choose to include more squatting, kneeling, crouching, etc. in the movements of your day. Look for opportunities to include more variety in your body positions. Do not overlook the opportunities to sit on the floor, kneel or crouch, etc.

Sitting and sleeping:
Choose to mechanically adjust your seats at work and in your car to alter your habitual manner of sitting, paying particular attention to your pelvic tilt.

At home, choose to use lumbar cushions as reminders to make a change from your habitual way of sitting.

Because my husband was spending a lot of time in the evening writing at his laptop computer, we bought a comfortable tilt seat bench with a table.

At night, he started sleeping on a memory foam mattress.

External stimuli:
Sometimes, during your day, choose to sit for short time periods on a heating pad or on different diameter and density of balls (tennis ball, T-ball).

Continue to stretch your "psoas" using "stretch psoas, leg hanging off the bed" and selected yoga postures (low lunge, up dog, bridge, pigeon with torso upright).

Felt senses of the body and pelvic pain:
Several times a day choose to practice **specifically focusing on felt senses** using full body scan or scan of specific areas of the

body. Choose to feature the body parts that may have linkages to the programmed pelvic pain. Choose to focus on sensations.

During your day while sitting, choose to tune into the felt senses of the tissues in your pelvis. Examine and experience how it feels at that moment – familiar or not, changing from moment to moment.

Sometime during the day choose to **practice a remembrance** of your pelvic pain. Tune into the area that you think the pain comes from and see if you can remember what it felt like – as many characteristics of the pain experience as you can recall. See if you can find where it was located in your body and remember what it felt like – intensity, duration, other characteristics. At that moment, consider if you can remember related feelings or sensations in other parts of your body (head, face, neck, shoulders, stomach, abdomen).

Thought content related to pelvic pain:
Working with thoughts associated with posture, position, and movement remains basically the same as described previously. Choose to feature thought content specific to the body, body movement, and pelvic pain.

Choose to address the thought reflexively with several comments or questions as described previously.

Thought content that is pelvic pain:
As best as you can, when you are having pelvic pain, redirect and distract reflexively with several comments or questions as described previously. *Do not answer your questions. Do not analyze or ruminate or elaborate.* Just silently ask the questions or make the comments:

- There is a thought about my pelvic pain.
- This is what the brain does. My brain contributes thoughts.
- What it contributes may not be useful or accurate.
- I, like other feeling entities, wish to be happy and to be free from pain.

Choose, *as best as you can,* to let go of whatever thought that has engaged your attention.

Choose to bring your attention back to what is happening in your day.

My husband *did not* use another option of working with the pain: to "attend" to the pain. Some believe that direct attention toward the pain can "de-bias" the system and interrupt the patterns that the brain is "stuck in.". There is not a lot of research to validate this point of view.

The research does suggest that having flexible attention and focusing skills influence the attentional bias away from being stuck in negative physical sensations (pain). Being "stuck" is a loss of freedom for your attention as the mind looks for the pain signals and ignores other information.

The work that my husband did is based on the belief that choosing to be an "observer" is more effective than confronting pain with an attitude of an "arm wrestler" or a "friend."

RESULTS

My husband began these practices (autonomic and somatic), training many systems at the same time and training using a variety of the exercises. He was always looking for opportunities, in his posture, changes in posture, movement, and other external and internal influences.

We were hopeful that he would find some relief, but the enormity of the outcome still leaves us amazed. He started these practices in June and was free from the pelvic pain by November. The issue of hesitancy continued to bother him.

5

Autonomic Control and Breath

Breathing is a function of our body that is done automatically, unconsciously (an autonomic function). It can also be controlled voluntarily, consciously. Research continues to suggest that the way we breathe decisively influences autonomic processing in many organ systems, including the urinary system, and that deep and voluntary, slow breathing practices can influence our involuntary functions.

ROLE OF THE AUTONOMIC SYSTEM

After a year of living pain-free, we were feeling most hopeful that the changes were promising to be permanent. My husband continued to choose opportunities throughout the day to practice working with physical posture, positions and movements. His practice of the basic drill for training attention and self-monitoring became less regular.

He continued to be bothered by his difficulty starting a urine stream (urinary hesitancy) day and night, many times accompanied by uncomfortable urethral spasm. His nocturia was consistent with his age.

We recognized that he was dealing with a function that is controlled by the autonomic nervous system (the inner sphincter function is controlled by the autonomic nervous system and is involuntary). We considered the relevant research on the autonomic nervous system and discovered much recent, promising research suggesting associations between chronic pelvic pain and differences in the autonomic nervous system *and* between the breath and the autonomic nervous system.

The mechanism of how "breathing interacts with the nervous system affecting metabolism and autonomic functions remains to be clearly understood. It is our hypothesis that voluntary slow, deep breathing functionally resets the autonomic nervous system." Ref: Jerath R, Edry JW, Barnes VA, Jerath V. Physiology of long pranayamic breathing: neural respiratory elements may provide a mechanism that explains how slow deep breathing shifts the autonomic nervous system. Med Hypotheses. 2006; 67(3): 566–71.

ADDITIONS TO THE READING LIST

Once my husband decided that working with his breath was an option that he wanted to explore, I went back to reading the research including research focused on:

> *voluntary slow, deep breathing and effects on the autonomic nervous system, mind-body skills for regulating the autonomic nervous system, breathing practices.*

I read as many scientific papers that I could find, trying to identify specifically what *instructions* were given in the clinical trials.

ADDITIONS TO THE PLAN

I outlined the additional practice goals:

5. Using his new skills, work in specific ways with his breath as another attention training exercise.
6. Using his new skills, work in specific ways to reacquaint his *body and brain* with his *breath* using diaphragmatic breathing through the nose.

Again the *plan* was simple. Do not try to force (arm wrestle) a change! Give his brain some new experiences, some redirection, and *get out of its way!*

INSTRUCTIONS FOR THE PRACTICE SEQUENCE OF VOLUNTARY, SLOW, DEEP BREATHING

I present this practice in the sequence that I suggested to my husband.

Sit in an easy, comfortable position maintaining good anatomical posture and consciously exhale to empty your lungs.

Acknowledge your intention to access the abilities of the body and brain.

Acknowledge your intention to maintain a consistent focus and consistent observation.

Voluntarily allow the focus of your attention and awareness to be on the sensations of your breath.

Consciously control an inhalation through your nose, filling your lungs from the bottom to the top during a slow count of six (6).

Choose to first contract the diaphragm with expansion of your "belly."

Choose to feel the movement of your ribs and intercostal muscles as they move upward and outward to allow the expansion of lung volume.

Pause for two (2) counts.

Control your exhalation through your nose, emptying from the bottom to the top with the slow count of six (6).

Pause for two (2) counts.

Repeat this cycle fifteen (15) times.

RESULTS

He started working with his breath without delay. He also returned to his daily practice of training attention skills and self-monitoring.

Within **two weeks,** the difficulty starting his urine stream (day and night) and the accompanying uncomfortable spasm had resolved.

Again, we had been hopeful that he would find some relief, but the resolution of this issue, sooner than we expected or hoped for, still leaves us amazed.

NOTE: **Choosing a breath practice.**

The instructions given in the clinical trials using breath-work as an intervention were "all over the place." There is a long history of breath-work techniques in spiritual and health practices, and the researchers had many theories of efficacy to choose from. As a result, there was little consistency in the instructions. Nevertheless, the practices chosen seem to consistently have the effect postulated with functions of the autonomic system.

I made the decision to start simple and teach something that I thought an American male would have the least resistance to – *a very short practice.* If this simple, short practice was not successful after a couple of months, I was prepared to recommend changes to the different variables – count, pace, total number of breaths, etc.

6

Last Thoughts

"It is a shame that we possess such insufficient knowledge concerning the character of pain—those symptoms which represent the essential part of all bodily suffering of man." Defter den Schmerz. Prof. Dr. A. Goldscheider. Berlin, 1894

WHY I WROTE THIS BOOK

Why did I write about this? I had not specifically examined my intentions until I started to struggle with writing an ending to this book. This is the first time I have seriously considered trying to contribute to a conversation about a problem that is ongoing and that affects so many lives.

The answer was that I felt that our successful experience might inspire others; that it might inspire hope.

I feel strongly:

- That the knowledge concerning the character of pain has been advanced.
- That the basics of pain science are very well accepted but generally ignored.

- That some percentage of the men experiencing chronic pelvic pain will find a resolution using this mind and body approach.

WHAT FORMAT?

I don't see myself as someone who buys and reads self-help books. But to be truthful, I have throughout my life gone to books, other printed matter, and the Internet for information to help my "self." This includes peeking into the lives of other people to understand how they confront challenges common in this human life.

My attitude has been, why try to reinvent the wheel? Why not use the experience and wisdom of others? Most of the time, I already had a foundation on which to build a solution or an understanding of an issue.

My use of self-help literature has not translated into an absolute understanding of how such a book should be organized to be of maximum benefit to a reader. My experiences influenced me in the following ways:

- I have tried to present this in an easy to read and follow manner.
- I have resisted my inclination to long, persuasion-themed discourses in favor of a bare recitation of the events.
- I have resisted using hype and jargon that often surrounds the explanation of training attention and awareness.
- I have resisted writing a scholarly, academic presentation.
- I have resisted writing a pathography.

LAST BUT NOT LEAST: THE ROLE OF INTENTION

I cannot emphasize enough the role that intention, the desire for relief, and the expectation of relief plays in "rewiring."

As we intentionally *choose* to shape our internal focus of attention in a particular manner, these strong subjective experiences, along with positive emotions, affect functional connections and also compete for allocation of our mental processing resources.

These mental processing resources are limited. Accordingly, the goal should be to provide more competition for the resources available for the processing and perception of information related to pelvic pain (mental or physical) by using the skills gained in training attention and by referencing positive personal intentions and expectations.

Practice:
Concepts and Suggestions

PRACTICE CONCEPTS

> *"concept" n. "an idea of what something is or how it works." Ref: "concept." Merriam Webster, 2014.* Merriam-Webster.com. *Web. 25 July 2014.*

FREQUENTLY REVIEWED CONCEPTS

Consistent with learning something new, my husband experienced "beginner's" uncertainty. He needed "reinforcing" information as he processed and acted on his new knowledge. He had to actively engage with the information (categorize, analyze, combine, reflect, conceptualize, synthesize, re-assess the value of the information, look for bias, omissions, etc.) and apply new understanding to his task of learning new skills. We reviewed and expanded concepts introduced previously.

Practice Concept: As Best You Can

This is one of the most important attitudes and intentions that should be cultivated. Whatever you choose to feature in your practice remember to do it "as best you can".

Accept that human struggle is a healthy part of life.

PRACTICE CONCEPT: Normal State Of Consciousness And Access To Thoughts

Humans experience different "states of consciousness". The state that I am addressing here is the level where we normally function when we are awake. We are not experiencing dreams, lucid dreams, hallucinations, transcendence, etc.

We are experiencing **normal conscious access** to **some of the results** of our brain activity. We are **aware**. We perceive. We observe the results in our "field of awareness".

I refer to brain results that we have conscious access to (awareness of, perception of) as "mental representations". Our brain has:

- Been stimulated internally or externally
- Processed the stimulus or stimuli
- Reached a "result" from the processing
- Shared **part** of the result in a particular way so that we have an experience of conscious access

The "mental representations" may also be referred to as "thoughts". Many of us refer to this as happening in our "mind". (I *try* to avoid using the term "mind" because it has too many subjective definitions that involve philosophical questions.)

Practice Concept: Relationship To Thoughts

1. What is our relationship to our thoughts?
Mental representations (thoughts) arising from our brain with
or without our effort typically are experienced and identified by
our "human self" as what "we know": *It comes from "my
mind/my brain" so it must be "me", it must be "true", etc.*

This can coexist with: *I am my "thoughts". The way my
mind works is just the way I am. I inherited some of the way my
mind works. The way I think makes me who I am. The way I
think makes me unique.*

We have not asked the questions:
Are these assumptions true? How did we get into this kind of
relationship with our mental representations? How did we get
into a relationship where the reactive mental processes of the
brain are in charge? How did we get into a relationship where
we are not in charge of our mental habits?

We have not asked the questions:
How did we get into a relationship that relies on such a *maladaptive* strategy? Is this the relationship that we want to be in?
Is this relationship beneficial? Do we want it to be a long-term
relationship? Are there other types of relationships that make
more sense?

The assumptions are probably not true. This is probably not
the most beneficial relationship that we could choose. We did
not get into this dysfunctional relationship by choice. We got
here by not understanding the design of our human body and
brain.

2. How did we learn this relationship to our thoughts?
Humans do not come with an operations manual with sections on:

- Human Body: Hardware and Software
- Human Brain: Choosing a Relationship to Your Thoughts

Imagine: you came into the world as a new model of computer with the latest hardware, the latest operating system, and the most excellent software for doing the work that you need to do. **What you also got was inadequate installation/initialization** of critical software for prevention of accidents or errors - to check for viruses, Trojan horses, malware, cultural memes, security issues, etc., and inadequate installation/initialization of your "fact checker" software.

As you have been living your life you connected to the internet of our culture. **Without the fully functional software**, you do not get a pop-up that asks: "This information is not from a source that you are familiar with and it may have problems with accuracy and ethics. Do you want to continue to download? If you say yes, you are also agreeing to allow our cookies." No pop-up that asks you: "Do you want to allow this to be downloaded onto your hard-drive, take up 14GB of your memory allocated in different places, and give you fits if you want to remove it." No pop-up that warns: "There is a problem completing that task or processing that normal request. You accept responsibility for the use of information as presented."

So as you try to get your work done here on earth **you experience the problems** like a computer that has been connected to the internet with no software for protection and with malfunctions in software:

- **You consistently come up with incorrect calculations in your "spreadsheets".**
- **You have failures that prevent you from finding or using historical files for making key decisions.**
- **You crash or freeze at inconvenient times.**

3. What happens in this kind of relationship?
Without an understanding of the brain design and without the fully functional software, humans will not get consistent, reliable use of the more recently developed parts of their brain which are valuable in:

- Checking facts
- Analyzing, comparing, evaluating
- Values clarification

These functions take place mostly out of the field of awareness!

The critical software is there. The problem is one of function: access and use. Because of human brain design we are able to train the brain, changing access and use. **Essential to training the brain is being in a proper relationship to thoughts.**

It is highly possible that some of the chronic pelvic pain problem is caused by incorrect calculations, lost files, and inaccessible files. It is possible that there is a problem of access and use.

In neural sensitization there are two ways this happens. A nerve that is repeatedly conducting sensory information to the brain about pain can become vulnerable so that it takes less and less of a trigger to result in the delivery of a greater and greater experience of pain. Sensitization can also occur at the level of the central nervous system, so that larger areas of the nervous system or even the whole body can become hyper-sensitive to stimulus, as well as hyper-reactive.

4. You can choose to cultivate the relationship of observer/witness.
The alternative relationship that I propose is one of **an observer, a witness who has knowledge, insight, and wisdom**. If you choose, you would affect the new relationship with practices in which you become familiar with what your brain is doing and how it works and in which you train some cognitive functions. (Even the act of acknowledging that you would prefer a different relationship, more in line with your values, is conducive to the change.)

In the practice of training attention, sustaining the feeling of being an observer/witness will change your relationship to your thoughts. You know that you are observing your own experience.

As you gain skill in sustaining this sense of being the observer, a space is opened between your "observer self" and the presentations from your brain (all thought that comes, with or without effort). Use this distance from your thoughts. Use effort, knowledge, insight, and wisdom to observe and evaluate what your brain is doing. Evaluate the activity and content of the thought representations for usefulness. Reappraise and problem solve. Make choices that serve your values.

The new relationship will also strengthen as you practice **sustaining the sense of being the observer throughout your daily life**, evaluating and choosing actions consistent with your values.

PRACTICE CONCEPT: Nonreactive Attitude, Being Judgmental, And Acceptance

1. Nonreactive attitude is not "acceptance of things as they are".
These practices may seem similar to meditation, "mindfulness", or mindfulness-based interventions. Research has shown these practices to be beneficial for humans in various physical and mental conditions.

The characteristics common in these interventions include a practice of:

- **Focused attention**, the voluntary focusing of attention on a chosen object, and
- **Open monitoring**, the voluntary focusing of attention on the content of experience and voluntary monitoring with a "nonreactive" attitude

Sometimes the "nonreactive" attitude has been described as "nonjudgmental". This has been interpreted by some to suggest "acceptance of things as they are", registering the facts observed without reacting to them in any way, without self-reference (I like, I dislike, etc.), judgment or reflection. This interpretation is widely accepted and used even though it fails to account for what happens cognitively or for what specific part of the practice allows life changing human cognitive transformations.

2. A more informed understanding of nonreactive attitude
A more useful understanding of "nonreactive" attitude would mean that in the observer relationship we would cultivate:

- An ability to observe without over-identifying with content
- An ability to observe and reflect without triggering habitual patterns of reacting in a disorganized, il-logical, emotional, and useless manner
- An ability to observe with openness, curiosity, and flexibility

3. A more informed understanding of being judgmental

Distinguishing *useful* from *not useful* mental representations requires evaluation and judgment.

Thoughts are either "useful" or "not useful" in getting the job done – our intended life's work, fulfillment of personal values.

- Useful thoughts – facilitate actions to long term goals, serve personal values (desirable to maximize the experience and their influence, desirable to acknowledge as useful, desirable to acknowledge the values that are served)
- Not useful thoughts – obstruct actions to long term goals, do not serve personal values (desirable to minimize the experience and their influence, de-sirable to acknowledge as not useful, desirable to acknowledge as obstruction to values)

In the observer/witness relationship, thoughts that are not use-ful are noted. They are targeted for untangling, dismantling, or examination.

4. Acceptances to cultivate

In the observer relationship we would cultivate an acceptance:

- **Of the way a human brain works**
- **Of the fact that we own a human brain**
- **Of the fact that we, as the "owner", have a responsibility**: To understand how our brain works, to use that understanding to be **in charge** of our brain, and to use that understanding to ensure that we are fulfilling our life's work

PRACTICE CONCEPT: Thoughts Come Without Effort Or With Effort

It is useful to recognize and acknowledge the way the brain works as it supplies content for our perception. This content that we are aware of (mental representations, mental objects, cognitive content) is presented in two ways:

1. Without effort: mental content appears without conscious exertion. It is automatic.
Initially when choosing to be the witness/observer there is a time (possibly very brief, fleeting) when we fix our attention on our breath or field of awareness with successful focus. Then suddenly we realize that what we are experiencing is NOT our chosen object of focus! It is some other content (aka mental object, cognitive content). We perceive content! We experience this as happening *without effort.*

Thoughts come, thoughts come, thoughts come! They come without effort.

Our attention engaged with the content may trigger the brain to follow-up with an automatic uncontrolled flow of mental events. Once the flow is started we perceive it running until completed, without any conscious effort, permission, direction, or guidance. The flow is not the chosen attention task. (Sometimes the engagement is **not in our field of awareness but can still trigger an automatic response**.)

2. With effort: mental content appears with conscious exertion. It is not automatic.
Once we experience our attention engaged with content we may follow-up with an earnest attempt to use mental abilities to

achieve something. It is intentional. We perceive the common activities of a normal human brain, which include analyzing, comparing, evaluating, planning, remembering, visualizing, etc. We are in charge of direction. We experience this as happening *with effort.*

The disadvantage of automatic processes: Our brain may develop habitual rigid maladaptive reactions. The flexibility to choose wisely is compromised. Because we are not consciously aware of the stimulus we cannot choose conscious regulation of reaction.

The advantage of automatic processes: It is an efficiency issue. We do not have to bring everything into our conscious field of awareness for consideration. We are not constantly challenged with exhaustion of our limited resources for executive attention and processing.

A simple example of this: Right versus wrong? We need an automatic reaction. We do not need to bring it into our field of awareness (unless it is a new or novel situation).

PRACTICE CONCEPT: Transformative Change

These practices allow life changing human cognitive transformations. Transformative change is likely made possible by doing work in two areas:

1. Internally focused cognitive work
Training of attention and awareness, body scans

- Develops a relationship to our thoughts that allows us distance to observe what our brain is doing, to evaluate content/activity for usefulness with our knowledge, insight, and wisdom, to identify content/activity that is not useful and needing examination
- Develops cognitive functions (used in **conscious** deliberations and in **unconscious** mental activity) that help us make sense of experiences

2. External cognitive work
Acquisition of information

- Increases our understanding of how our human brain/body works so that we may use it in the way it is designed

Cognitive work on content/mental activity that we have identified as not being useful and as needing examination: Professional help may be required for adequate progress.

- Untangles dysfunctional wiring
- Dismantles dysfunctional stories

"Wisdom work"

- Clarifies values through self reflection
- Clarifies values through prioritizing value driven activities (religious, social, friendship, family, citizenship, student, etc.) from our historical cultures

Because of the possibility of transformative change, this attention skill can be used not just for health but also for all areas of life. Using this skill facilitates transition in self-statements:

- From: "I am…" or "I feel…"
- To: "I am currently experiencing sensations / representations that are commonly labeled…."

Both internally and externally focused cognitive work is **required** if we wholeheartedly desire change!

PRACTICE CONCEPT: What You Resist Will Persist.

It appears that the brain ironically cannot always tell itself what to do.

The deliberate attempt to suppress worrying thoughts about pelvic pain will make them more likely to surface in your field of awareness. Because of the "ironic process", what you attempt to resist will only persist.

I encourage avoidance of using effort to "force things from my mind".

I encourage avoidance of using self-statements such as: "I will not do that."

PRACTICE CONCEPT: Inward Focus Of Attention (Interoceptive, Internally Focused)

Ways to focus the attention inward:

- Focus attention on breath sensations or field of awareness during the practice of training attention
- Scan/inventory of the entire body for sensations
- Specific scan of pelvic area for sensations
- Specific scan of other body parts that may have connections to pelvic pain (postural, hip and leg)
- Practice of a "remembrance" of pelvic pain

Use of internally focused attention is encouraged for two reasons.

- These interoceptive (internally focused) attention practices use more evolutionarily older parts of the brain that are likely associated with sensation and integration of physical experience.
- In the parasympathetic system, the spinal cord directly innervates body parts. It is likely that neural activity increases in the spinal segment innervating the body area that is being "attended" to in a body scan.

Practice Concept: Using Habitual Reflexive Response

The reason to use the same reflexive responses (acknowledge with the same simple comments, redirect with predetermined distraction) is because you want the most efficacious action when an opportunity arises.

The intention of the response is already defined. The initiation of the response can be immediate when it has been practiced to the point that it becomes "reflexive".

I strongly recommend using these three specific comments to "Acknowledge":

- There is a thought (about my pelvic pain).
- This is what the brain does. My brain contributes thought.
- What it contributes may not be useful or accurate.

Practice Concept: Contributions From Other Life Experiences

During this time you are working, writing papers, editing papers, preparing lectures, teaching, playing guitar, learning music theory, following current events and other subjects that hold your interest, and occasionally making time for daydreaming. At the same time, I am sharing what I am reading and learning especially about neuroplasticity and training the brain.

I cannot discount that this (a steady diet of new information and discussions, the use of your analytical and critical thinking functions, the down-time of daydreaming) plays a role in the changes you experience.

Practice Support (PS)

> "support" n. "the act of helping someone by giving love, encouragement, etc.." Ref: "support." Merriam Webster, 2014. Merriam-Webster.com. Web. 25 July 2014.

I offered support to my husband as he worked to hone his attention and awareness skills and as he worked in specific ways with his thought and emotions.

The following daily practice suggestions for attention were constructed to offer clarification in response to the questions that came up as he started learning these new skills.

The suggestions for work with the body emphasize:

- Posture
- "Everything is a squat."
- Tiny changes
- Scan of body, pelvic area
- Felt senses
- Choosing to thoughtfully construct and use if (when)/then action plans
- "As best you can."

PS1 Intention

Mental:

Begin your practice by acknowledging your intention to access the abilities of the body and brain.

Acknowledge your intention to maintain a consistent focus and consistent observation of your breath.

Recognize when your attention wanders, *note that it has wandered, choose to let go of whatever has engaged the attention without judgment, discourse, or rumination* and choose to bring your attention back to the breath sensations.

> *Remember: It is not necessary to examine the content of the distractions at this time.*

Body:

Sometimes today choose to *"take an inventory"* of your standing body posture. Begin with you feet and work your way up your body, noting your habitual default posture. Specifically choose to change position in two areas: Shoulder blades and pelvis.

PS2 Posture For Practice

Mental:

A comfortable sitting position, maintaining good anatomical posture, can be achieved on the floor or in a chair. Position your hands comfortably. There is no particular way of doing this. Just try to keep your hands in a way that enhances your comfort and relaxation. If you experience any discomfort, make adjustments to relieve the discomfort. If you have an itch, scratch it. Practicing in a quiet location can be useful but not mandatory.

Body:

Sometimes today choose to *"take an inventory"* of your sitting body posture. Can you feel that you are on your "sitting bones"? Choose to make a *tiny*, conscious change in your pelvic tilt.

PS3 Normal Brain

Mental:

When observing your breath it may seem that your attention is drawn to something else more often than it is following the breath. This is normal activity for the brain. As you have more practice experience you will have times that you feel your attention is stable on your breath. Other times you will experience that it is less stable, that your attention is taking side trips at every moment. You are not unique! This is what everyone (even people with thousands of hours of practice) reports. Welcome to exploring the world of your brain.

> *Note the side trip and choose to let go without judgment, discourse, or rumination.* Choose to bring your attention back to the breath sensations.

Body:

Sometimes today choose to pause before you sit down. Choose to purposefully make the action of sitting the specific "down" motion of a "squat".

PS4 Tradition

Mental:

In training attention, choosing to focus on the breath is tradi-
tional and convenient.

Body:

Sometimes today choose to pause before you come from a sitting
position to a standing position. Choose to purposefully make the
action of standing the specific "up" motion of a "squat".

PS5 Comparing

Mental:

It is not necessary or useful to compare your practice to that of another day or to that of another person. Choose an attitude and intention of compassion.

Acknowledge your intention to maintain a consistent focus and consistent observation. Acknowledge that as you practice attending your breath, whatever happens is part of the practice and is useful. If your attention wanders to something else, *note that it has wandered, choose to let go of whatever has engaged the attention without judgment, discourse, or rumination* and choose to bring your attention back to the breath sensations.

Body:

Sometime today choose to take time to use a full-length mirror to review your posture with reference to anatomical position. Evaluate: feet are hip distance apart, equal external rotation of feet and legs, knees equally flexed and extended with no hyper-flexion, hip points level, length in your spine, ears over shoulders, shoulder blades toward the middle of the back and down slightly, belly button awareness with a slight movement towards the spine.

Choose to make tiny, conscious changes in what has been your default posture.

PS6 Flowing Stream Of Thoughts

Mental:

Recognize when distracting mental representations (thoughts, mind wandering) are numerous and persistent (like rush hour traffic or flowing of a stream), causing your attention to be distracted from your chosen object of attention – your breath. *Note the flow and choose to let go without judgment, discourse, or rumination.* Choose to bring your attention back to the breath sensations.

Body:

Sometimes today, **specifically** choose to make a *tiny*, conscious change in your pelvic tilt.

PS7 Therapy

Mental:

As with any physical therapy, more progress is achieved by practicing a small amount of time every day than by practicing a longer amount time less frequently.

There is no value in chastising yourself when a practice is missed.

Body:

Sometimes during this day, choose a time when you will be changing from a sitting position to a standing position. Pause for a moment to "take an inventory" of your posture, noting an area that you have identified for attention. Make *tiny* adjustments.

PS8 Values And Intentions

Mental:

Begin your practice with a reference to your positive personal intentions and expectations, the desire to live a life skillfully accomplishing your life's work. Acknowledge this as your real reason for doing this practice.

Without force, sustain the feeling of being the observer.

Recognize when your attention wanders, *note that it has wandered, choose to let go of whatever has engaged the attention without judgment, discourse, or rumination* and choose to bring your attention back to the breath sensations.

> *Remember: It is not necessary to examine the content of the distractions at this time.*

Body:

Sometimes during your day when sitting, see if you can feel that you are on your "sitting bones." Choose to make a *tiny*, conscious change in your pelvic tilt.

PS9 Without Force

Mental:

Monitor, without force, to sustain your focus on the breath.

Recognize when your attention wanders, *note that it has wandered, choose to let go of whatever has engaged the attention without judgment, discourse, or rumination* and choose to bring your attention back to the breath sensations.

Body:

Sometimes during your day, choose to specifically tune in to your walking motions, on flat surfaces or when climbing stairs. Choose, when you start to walk, to tune in to the feeling of lifting your leg using your hip flexor muscles, feeling your leg swing forward from your hip. Feel your heel touch the ground, and then the movement of your ankle as the sole of your foot and then the toes make the connection for push-off (heel-sole-toe). Feel the rotation (internal/external) of your leg (thigh, knee and feet should be same).

PS10 Choose

Mental:

There are other sensations that you experience during breathing –expansion of chest volume, movement of belly, etc.

In your practice voluntarily choose to allow the focus of your attention to be on the inhalational sensations of your breath (cooler air flowing into your nostrils, warming as it flows through the nasal cavity) and then the exhalational sensations of the warmed air.

Body:

As you look for opportunities to include more variety in your body positions, choose to sit on the floor. Explore to find an activity on the floor that you can frequently find useful and enjoyable.

PS11 Consistent

Mental:

Breathe normally through your nose – no breath manipulation. Acknowledge your intention to maintain a consistent focus and consistent observation of your breath.

Recognize when your attention in distracted by the sensations of sound. *Note that it has wandered, choose to let go of whatever has engaged the attention without judgment, discourse, or rumination* and choose to bring your attention back to the breath sensations.

Body:

Sometimes during your day when you are lying down, choose to specifically *"take an inventory"* of your body. With this inventory, feature felt sensations. Briefly note the quality, intensity or other characteristics of the felt sensation.

Begin at your feet and move up your body with your examination – feet, ankle, calf, knee, thigh, hips, buttocks, pelvic area, abdomen, spine, chest, back, shoulders, upper arm, lower arm, hand, neck, face and head.

PS12 Observer

Mental:

Acknowledge that you are choosing to monitor your mental representations of your breath, without force.

Acknowledge that you are choosing to sustain, without force, the feeling of being the **observer** - observing your breath and observing when you are distracted.

Recognize when distracting thoughts are numerous and persistent. *Note the spontaneous flow and choose to let go without judgment, discourse, or rumination.* Choose to bring your attention back to the breath sensations.

Body:

Sometimes during your day, choose to specifically tune in to your movements as you start to sit in your chair at your desk, in the seat of the car, etc. Pause for a moment to "take an inventory" of your posture, choosing to specifically target the feeling of **your pelvic position**. Choose to make a *tiny*, conscious change in your pelvic tilt.

PS13 Self-Monitoring And Directing Attention

Mental:

Practice exercises are initially intended to *train and strengthen your ability to monitor* for where your attention is. The "self-monitoring" functional area of the brain is trainable.

Bringing the attention back to the breath begins the *training for the skill of directing* your attention, of *strengthening your ability to place your attention* on an object of your choice.

Body:

Sometimes during your day, choose to specifically tune in to your movements as you start to sit (in your chair at your desk, in the seat of the car, etc.) pause for a moment to "take an inventory" your posture, choosing to specifically target the feeling of your **hip flexor movement**. Focus on the felt sensations. Choose to make a *tiny*, conscious change in your movement.

PS14 Skills

Mental:

> "...the ability to focus and sustain attention on an intended object requires skills involved in monitoring the focus of attention and detecting distraction, disengaging attention from the source of distraction, and (re)directing and engaging attention to the intended object." Ref: Lutz A, Slagter HA, Dunne J, Davidson RJ. *Attention regulation and monitoring in meditation.* Trends Cogn. Sci. 2008; 12: 163–169.

Without force, sustain the feeling of being the observer.

Recognize your ability to focus and sustain attention on your intended object: your breath. Recognize your skill in monitoring and detecting distraction when your attention wanders in distraction. Recognize your skill as you *note that it has wandered, you choose to disengage with the source of distraction without judgment, discourse, or rumination* and you choose to distract, redirect, and bring your attention back to your intended object, your breath sensations.

Body:

Sometimes during your day, choose to specifically tune in to your movements. When you start to stand up, or you start to sit (in your chair at your desk, in the seat of the car, etc.), pause for a moment to "take an inventory" of your posture. Recognize that these movements are "squats".

PS15 Monitoring Your Field Of Awareness

Mental:

The brain contributes mental representations (thoughts) into our "field of awareness".

Monitor and observe all of your mental activity presenting in the field of awareness, much the same as you imagine that you are standing on the command deck of a spaceship hurtling through deep space as you observe the space debris, shooting stars, and other spaceships that streak into your view and continue out of your sight into the darkness of space.

As you choose to feature the sense of being an observer, focus your attention on your field of view that is being populated with information picked up by all of your sensory organs (smell, taste, touch, hearing, somatic, visceral, proprioceptions) and the results of the processing of the stimuli (including your responses...with and without effort). As best you can, choose not to engage with the content.

Body:

Sometimes during your day while sitting, choose to tune into the felt senses of the tissues in your pelvis. Examine and experience how it feels at that moment – familiar or not, changing from moment to moment.

PS16 Different Relationship

Mental:

This early practice is for strengthening the attention "muscle" and is not for working with content.

The practice is a monitoring of the display of what is occurring, observing the streams of content without engaging. It is a practice of a different relationship to what is arising in your field of awareness - that of an observer of your own experience.

Recognize when your attention wanders, *note that it has wandered, choose to let go of whatever has engaged the attention without judgment, discourse, or rumination* and choose to skillfully bring your attention back to monitoring and observing your field of awareness.

Choosing to put your attention where you want it to be strengthens your skills and strengthens the new relationship.

Body:

Sometimes during your day when standing, see if you can feel the position of your pelvis. Choose to make a *tiny*, conscious change in your pelvic tilt, slightly changing the tilt of your pelvis.

PS17 Appears Without Effort

Mental:

Observe all of your mental activity in the field of awareness. Some appear without effort. Some appear after you choose to be in charge, using some effort to determine the direction of your conscious cognition. Appreciate how this activity can be observed as it passes through your field of awareness.

Recognize when your attention wanders, *note that it has wandered, choose to let go of whatever has engaged the attention without judgment, discourse, or rumination* and choose to bring your attention back to monitoring your field of awareness.

Body:

Sometimes during your day when sitting, see if you can feel that you are on your "sitting bones." Briefly "take an inventory" for the position of your shoulder blades. Make tiny adjustments. Imagine that you are lengthening your spine, creating more space between your vertebrae.

PS18 Senses

Mental:

As you choose to increase the feeling of being an observer, focus your attention on your field of view that is being populated with information picked up by all of your sensory organs (smell, taste, touch, hearing, somatic, visceral, proprioceptions).

This practice of the "being an observer" will transform your relationship to your "thoughts". You are NOT your thoughts.

Body:

Sometimes during your day, choose to specifically tune in to your walking motions, on flat surfaces or when climbing stairs. Choose, when you start to walk, to tune in to the feeling of lifting your leg using your hip flexor muscles, feeling your leg swing forward from your hip. Feel your heel touch the ground, and then the movement of your ankle as the sole of your foot and then the toes make the connection for push-off (heel-sole-toe). Feel the rotation (internal/external) of your leg (thigh, knee and feet should be same).

PS19 Good Practice

Mental:

It is natural for your brain to offer congratulations to you on days that it concludes you are having "a good practice". This certainty or feelings of conviction or rightness isn't within your conscious control. It is another result of your brain using recent input, recent memory, and long-term memory to present you with results of an analysis. This is another opportunity to practice a different relationship to the thought.

Choose to let go of whatever congratulatory thought that has engaged your attention. Choose to bring your attention back to monitoring your field of awareness.

Body:

Sometimes during your day when you must "pick up" an object, consider your options – "bending over" or making the movement a squat.

Choose to make the movement a squat. Focus on the felt sensations in your pelvic area.

PS20 Engaged In Monitoring

Mental:

Acknowledge your intention to practice "self monitoring": to maintain a consistent focus of attention on your field of awareness and to maintain a consistent sense of being the observer of the activity in your field.

Acknowledge that mental representations can come without effort.

Recognize when distracting thoughts are numerous and persistent. *Note the spontaneous flow and choose to let go without judgment, discourse, or rumination.* Choose to bring your attention back to your field of awareness.

Body:

Sometimes during your day while sitting, choose to do a body scan. Focus on the qualities of the felt sensations from each body part. Imagine "breathing" a relaxation into areas that appear to be reporting tension.

PS21 Feature The Sense

Mental:

Choose to feature the feeling of being an observer as you engage in monitoring your field of awareness - your field of view that is being populated with information picked up by all of your sensory organs (smell, taste, touch, hearing, somatic, visceral, proprioceptions).

The observer *"monitors"* what is coming into your field of awareness. Choose not to engage with the content.

Body:

Sometimes during your day when standing, tune into the sensations in your pelvic area as you make *tiny*, conscious changes in your posture.

PS22 Strengthen The *New* Relationship

Mental:

Be confident that both "mind wandering" and "mind engaging in monitoring" are part of the practice drill. Both are useful in accomplishing your goal.

Acknowledge your choice to engage in self-monitoring.

Choose to cultivate the perception of being an observer. This strengthens the new relationship to your thoughts.

Body:

Choose to feature your standing body posture.

Choose to *"take an inventory"* of your standing body posture. Begin with you feet and work your way up your body, noting your habitual default posture. Specifically choose to change position in two areas: shoulder blades and pelvis.

PS23 Observe Not Control

Mental:

Recognize when distracting thoughts or sensations are numerous and persistent. It is not necessary nor is it desirable to use effort, to try to control the kinds of representations that you experience in your field. You are a **witness** observing your inner world.

> *Note the spontaneous flow and choose to let go without judgment, discourse, or rumination.*

Body:

Today choose to feature your sitting body posture.

Choose to *"take an inventory"* of your sitting body posture. Can you feel that you are on your "sitting bones"? Choose to make a *tiny*, conscious change in your pelvic tilt.

PS24 Skills Not Content

Mental:

There will be themes to the content that you observe. At this time choose to emphasize the skill of attention and awareness and the practice of a new relationship. Working with content is addressed at another time.

Recognize when your attention wanders, *note that it has wandered, choose to let go of whatever has engaged the attention without judgment, discourse, or rumination* and choose to bring your attention back to monitoring your field of awareness.

Body:

Today choose to feature sitting and "everything is a squat".

Choose to pause before you sit down. Choose to purposefully make the action of sitting the specific "down" motion of a "squat".

PS25 Traffic

Mental:

Observe all of your mental activity in the field of awareness, much the same as you would look out a window of your house and observe the traffic as it goes by and continues down the street until it is out of sight.

> *This specific practice is for strengthening the attention "muscle" and does not work with content.*

Body:

Choose to feature standing up and "everything is a squat".

Choose to pause before you come from a sitting position to a standing position. Choose to purposefully make the action of standing the specific "up" motion of a "squat".

PS26 Observe Inner World

Mental:

The brain contributes mental representations into your "field of awareness". No one else has access to this - **your** inner world. You are the only one who can observe it.

As you choose to be an observer of your inner world, focus your attention on your field of awareness.

This field of view is being populated as your brain responds to the information picked up by **all** of your sensory organs (smell, taste, touch, hearing, somatic, visceral, proprioception) with an "analysis" and "conclusion".

"Monitor" what is coming into your field of awareness. Choose not to engage with the content. Choose the new relationship.

Body:

Today choose to feature posture: feet are hip distance apart, equal external rotation of feet and legs, knees with no hyperflexion, length in your spine, ears over shoulders, shoulder blades position, belly button awareness.

Choose to make tiny, conscious changes in what has been your default posture.

PS27 Breath

Mental:

As you sit in observation on a particularly busy day in the field of awareness, you may find it useful to return to the basic first part of practicing "attention to breath".

Body:

Choose to feature standing up.

When changing from a siting position to a standing position, pause for a moment. "Take an inventory" of your posture, noting an area that you have identified for attention. Make *tiny* adjustments.

PS28 Effort And Reason

Mental:

This practice requires effort. Effort is required in the learning of any new information or skill.

Acknowledge that your commitment and action in practice is consistent with your positive personal intentions and expectations, the desire to live a life skillfully accomplishing your life's work. Acknowledge this as your real reason for doing this practice.

Body:

Today choose to feature your movements as you start to sit in your chair at your desk, in the seat of the car, etc. Pause for a moment to "take an inventory" of your posture, choosing to specifically target the feeling of **your pelvic position**. Choose to make a *tiny*, conscious change in your pelvic tilt.

PS29 Human Discomfort

Mental:

This practice is at first **unfamiliar** as you:

1) Learn where your attention is and
2) Strengthen the ability to direct and place your attention on your object of choice (breath or field of awareness).

It may bring feelings of **discomfort**.

This is an opportunity for practice also.

Observe that this discomfort has engaged your attention. Acknowledge that humans experience discomfort. Choose to let go and to bring your attention back to observing your field of awareness.

Body:

Choose to feature your movements as you start to sit in your chair at your desk, in the seat of the car, etc. Pause for a moment to "take an inventory" of your posture, choosing to specifically target the feeling of **your hip flexor movement**. Choose to make a *tiny*, conscious change in your pelvic tilt.

PS30 Work With Content

Mental:

During your sitting practice begin to note content and themes of content in a general way.

To work with the observed content of your thoughts (those presenting with or without effort), use a 2-part response:

- **Acknowledge** with simple comments: There is a thought. This is what the brain does. My brain contributes random thoughts. What it contributes may not be useful.

- **Redirect**: Choose to bring your attention back to observing your field of awareness.

Body:

Sometimes during your day while sitting, choose to tune into the felt senses of the tissues in your pelvis. Examine and experience how it feels at that moment – familiar or not, changing from moment to moment, the qualities of the sensations.

PS31 Practice New Relationship

Mental:

Choose to feature the sense of being an observer of content in your inner world, focusing your attention on your field of awareness.

Observe the content. Often there will be themes to the content. Choose to address what you are noting with the same simple comments or questions. *Do not answer your questions. Do not analyze or ruminate or elaborate. Choose to let go of whatever thought has engaged your attention without judgment, discourse, or rumination.*

Choose to practice your new relationship.

Acknowledge:
There is a thought. This is what the brain does. My brain contributes random thoughts. What it contributes may not be useful.

Redirect:
Choose to bring your attention back to observing your field of awareness.

Body:

Today choose to feature the position of your pelvis. Choose to make a *tiny*, conscious change in your pelvic tilt, slightly changing the tilt of your pelvis.

PS32 No Access To Origin

Mental:

Common processes of a normal human brain include analyzing, comparing, evaluating, planning, remembering, visualizing. Most of these deliberations are not taking place in your field of awareness. Most are not within your conscious control.

The results of your brain processing recent input, recent memory, and long-term memory **can appear** in your field of awareness. **You don't have access to where the representation came from, where it was before it reached your field awareness.**

This is opportunity to practice a different relationship to the observed thought. Acknowledge that you do not have access to the origin of thoughts within your field of awareness. Acknowledge that you can witness the results.

Body:

Today choose to feature the position of your shoulder blades. Make tiny adjustments. Imagine that you are lengthening your spine, creating more space between your vertebrae.

PS33 Two-Parts

Mental:

To work with the content of your mental representations in a general way, recognize when you no longer sustain the feeling of being a witness. Recognize that you have engaged with content. Choose to address this in two parts:

Acknowledge:
There is a thought. This is what the brain does. My brain contributes random thoughts. What it contributes may not be useful.

Redirect:
Choose to bring your attention back to observing your field of awareness.

Body:
Choose to feature your "sitting bones."

PS34 Simple

Mental:
Cognitive changes will happen with simple responses.

Acknowledge:
There is a thought. This is what the brain does. My brain contributes random thoughts. What it contributes may not be useful.

Redirect:
Choose to bring your attention back to observing your field of awareness.

Body:
Today choose to feature walking motions.

Choose, when you start to walk, to tune in to the feeling of lifting your leg using your hip flexor muscles, feeling your leg swing forward from your hip. Feel your heel touch the ground, and then the movement of your ankle as the sole of your foot and then the toes make the connection for push-off (heel-sole-toe). Feel the rotation (internal/external) of your leg (thigh, knee and feet should be same).

PS35 Reflexive, Same Script

Mental:

Cognitive changes in self-monitoring activities facilitate the ability to **reflexively identify** that your attention has been distracted. They enable you to have a **reflexive response**.

Choose to use the same simple script for your response.

Acknowledge:

There is a thought. This is what the brain does. My brain contributes random thoughts. What it contributes may not be useful or accurate.

Redirect:

Choose to bring your attention back to observing your field of awareness.

Body:

Choose to feature the felt sensations in your pelvic area.

PS36 Different Relationship, Different Conclusions

Mental:

One goal of this practice with your attention and your field of awareness is to change the fundamental relationship that you have with your thoughts and mental representations.

With your improved skills you gain the ability (and a "space") to perceive transient mental events as objects to be observed. This change in relationship facilitates cognitive **activities** in your brain to arrive at a different conclusion with respect to your symptoms.

These common **activities** of a normal human brain include analyzing, comparing, evaluating, planning, remembering, visualizing. Most of these cognitive deliberations are **not taking place in your field of awareness**.

Body:

Today choose to feature standing. Tune into the sensations in your pelvic area as you make *tiny*, conscious changes in your posture.

PS37 Content Is About Pelvic Pain

Mental:

During your sitting practice, begin to note content and themes of content that are about pelvic pain.

To work with the content of your thoughts and emotions that are specifically about pelvic pain, choose to note the content using specific refutations, redirections, or comments.

Choose to use the same simple script for your response.

Acknowledge:

There is a thought with connections to my pelvic pain. This is what the brain does. My brain contributes thoughts. What it contributes may not be useful or accurate.

Redirect:

I, like other feeling entities, wish to be happy and to be free from pain. I choose to bring my attention back to observing my field of awareness.

> *You do not need to address the content more specifically in this basic drill.*

Body:

Choose to feature posture.

PS38 Simple

Mental:

Keep it simple. This *is* the basic drill for training attention skill.

Choose to be an observer of your field of awareness, your field of view that is being populated by the brain after it processes information picked up by all of your sensory organs (smell, taste, touch, hearing, somatic, visceral, proprioceptions).

From an observer relationship, monitor your field and your mental activity that arises within your field of awareness.

No one else has access to the world you carry around within yourself.

Body:

Choose to feature felt senses of the tissues in your pelvis. Examine and experience how it feels at that moment – familiar or not, changing from moment to moment, the qualities of the sensations.

PS39 Right Practice

Mental:

How am I doing? Am I doing this right? Is my mind too busy?

The intention of the practice is not the cessation of brain activity. It is not about repressing thoughts or content of thought. The practice is simply a drill

- To **improve your skills** of monitoring and redirection
- To **change your relationship** to your thoughts
- To **change cognitive functions** related to your pelvic pain
- To **change neural functions** related to your pelvic pain

Choose to remember that your brain contributes evaluations into your field of awareness. Choose to address content with your reflexive comments.

Acknowledge:

There is a thought. This is what the brain does. My brain contributes thoughts. What it contributes may not be useful or accurate.

Redirect:

I, like other feeling entities, wish to be happy and to be free from pain. I choose to bring my attention back to observing my field of awareness.

Body:

Today choose to feature postural position of your pelvis.

PS40 Busy Day

Mental:

As you sit in observation on a particularly "busy" day out there in your field of awareness, you may find it useful to briefly check into your felt sense of the body. In a **brief body scan** note perception of felt sensation of tension (another mental representation of what is happening in your body).

Acknowledge that the tension is a thought:
There is a thought. This is what the brain does. My brain contributes thoughts. What it contributes may not be useful or accurate.

Redirect:
Choose to breath a relaxation into the areas involved before returning to practicing "attention to breath".

Body:

Choose to feature your walking motions, on flat surfaces or when climbing stairs. Choose, when you start to walk, to tune in to the feeling of lifting your leg using your hip flexor muscles, feeling your leg swing forward from your hip. Feel your heel touch the ground, and then the movement of your ankle as the sole of your foot and then the toes make the connection for push-off (heel-sole-toe). Feel the rotation (internal/external) of your leg (thigh, knee and feet should be same).

PS41 Switch Focus

Mental:

As you sit in observation on a particularly "busy" day out there in your field of awareness you may find it useful to switch between focus options during your practice. As you learn the changing nature of your field of awareness, you may find it useful:

- To return to the basic practicing attention to breath.
- To observe the content without engaging.
- To observe the content with engaging.

If you engage, your reflexive response has 2 parts.

Acknowledge:
There is a thought. This is what the brain does. My brain contributes random thoughts. What it contributes may not be useful or accurate.

Redirect:
I, like other feeling entities, wish to be happy and to be free from pain. I choose to bring my attention back to observing my field of awareness.

Body:

Today choose to feature the feeling of lifting your leg using your hip flexor muscles.

PS42 Consistent, Frequent

Mental:

Familiarity with the changing nature of your field of awareness comes with the consistency of frequent practice. It is helpful to maintain an attitude of curiousness and openness.

It is not necessary to address the content more specifically in this basic drill. The skills acquired will be **used throughout your day** to untangle the pelvic pain programed into posture, movements, thoughts and emotions.

Body:

Today choose to feature "sitting".

PS43 Wandering

Mental:

You experience "mind wandering":

- Content "appearing without effort" as you are sucked into a habitual story without your permission
- Content you have chosen "effort" as a response, (engage and pursue the content with planning, ruminating, analyzing, examining, etc.)

Acknowledge what is happening as:
- Without effort
- With effort

Redirect.

Body:

Choose to feature felt sensations in your pelvic area. Observe that these sensations are within your field of awareness as a result of the processing activities of your brain. There may be errors.

PS44 Triggers

Mental:

Choose to acknowledge when your mind is mind wandering. Acknowledge that you can be "triggered" by the content to slide into a sequence of thoughts, a habitual story.

Practice a new and different relationship to your thoughts by **choosing** to redirect.

Body:

Today choose to feature equal external rotation of feet and legs.

PS45 Work With Your Thoughts Throughout Your Day

Mental:

The basic drill work gives you skills to work with content at any time so that you may change the relationship to your thoughts in your daily life.

Change is facilitated when you choose to work with your thought and emotion content throughout your day.

Most times it is sufficient to use Limited Examination. Choose to address what you are observing with the same simple, reflexive comments or questions. *Do not answer your questions. Do not analyze or ruminate or elaborate.* Choose to let go of whatever thought has engaged your attention and to bring your attention back to what is happening in your day.

Other times you may recognize the need for more in-depth Examination. Acknowledge that a recurring thought or emotional content observed is a major contribution to the maintenance of your pelvic pain. Acknowledge that your best choice would be to choose to do conscious cognitive work at another time. Options for conscious cognitive work include self-help, group work in a community of your choice, and *professional help.*

Body:

Today choose to feature belly button awareness.

PS46 Cultivating Solutions

Mental:

You want your brain to excel in **creative problem solving**. Creativity involves the use of different functional areas of the brain and of diversity in interactions between those areas.

It requires recruiting many areas critical for daydreaming, imagining the future, remembering deeply personal memories, reflecting constructively, making sense of experience, and processing social information.

It requires networking the areas and instigating many interacting cognitive processes (both conscious and unconscious).

This is achievable because the human brain is plastic - its structure and function change in response to experience.

Body:

Sometimes during this day choose a time to "take an inventory" of your posture, noting an area that **you** have identified for attention. Make *tiny* adjustments.

PS47 Allocation Of Resources

Mental:

The spontaneous representations from your brain are based on YOUR LIFE. The "stories" that get repeated often are the ones that have had the most support (allocation of your brain resources) in your past.

Two ways the story is supported:

- You choose to support it through your efforts of thinking, planning, ruminating, etc.
- You choose to let your brain support it when you consent to habitual, unchecked thought.

Either way, our brain will be an expert in replaying the stories unless you choose to become more involved in allocation of resources.

Training attentional resources allow you to become skillfully involved as opportunity arises.

Choose to work with your thought and emotion content throughout your day.

Acknowledge. Redirect.

Body:

Today choose to feature an action plan specific to your schedule today.

PS48 Scarce Resources

Mental:

The brain has to allocate its resources like the "brain real estate" (the physical structures including the habituated connections, a.k.a. the wiring) **and** the "executive functions" (required to maintain the real estate).

Ideally, resources would preferentially be devoted to habitual patterns that are **supportive of your values**. Ideally, resources would preferentially be devoted to habitual mind/body relationships that are **supportive of your health**.

The attention practices have as one objective a more skillful management of the allocation of these resources, some of them **scarce resources**.

Training and using your attentional skills affects:

- Skillful allocation that you can observe within your field of awareness as you choose to use effort and be involved.
- Skillful allocation **not within you ability to observe**.

Body:

Practicing functional anatomical alignment supports a habit of a "sustainable" posture.

PS49 Functional Areas Of Brain

Mental:

Different functional areas of your brain are involved in the maintenance of these stories of your life.

Choose activities that will require dynamic interaction of the different functional areas of your brain where memories are stored. Think of it as **instigating a reshuffling of your "deck"** so that the result is a new "hand of cards" critical for cultivating a solution.

Limited Examination: Choose to address what you are observing with simple comments or questions.

Examination: Acknowledge that a recurring thought or emotional content observed is part of the contribution by your brain to the programming of your pelvic pain. Choose self-help. Choose to work on your wisdom. Choose to examine your history with a *professional.*

Body:

Practicing anatomical alignment uses many functional areas of the brain.

PS50 Provide Opportunities

Mental:

Pelvic pain is likely to contain many **errors** in neural processing.

Provide lots of information and lots of opportunity for your brain and other neural tissues to avoid or correct errors and to initiate the desired action.

Throughout your day choose to work in specific ways with your thought and emotion content and with physical posture, position and movement that are part of the pelvic pain complex.

Use the space provided by a new relationship with your thoughts. Choose to be in charge of your mental habits.

Acknowledge. Redirect.

Body:

Sometime during the day choose to **practice a remembrance** of your pelvic pain. Tune into the area that you think the pain comes from and see if you can remember what it felt like – as many characteristics of the pain experience as you can recall: where it was located in your body, what it felt like – intensity, duration, other characteristics.

PS51 Practice New Relationship

Mental:

Throughout your day choose to work in specific ways with your thought and emotion content.

In the moment that you observe content that is not useful in helping you achieve your life's work, you can acknowledge that you made no effort with this mental representation.

Practice your new relationship. Acknowledge that you had no control over it appearing at this moment. Choose to redirect your attention to objects of your choice.

Body:

Feature the sense of being a witness to the feeling of lifting your leg using your hip flexor muscles, feeling your leg swing forward from your hip.

PS52 Choice

Mental:

In the moment that you observe content that is not useful in helping you achieve your life's work, you can acknowledge that you have exercised a choice in this mental representation.

Choice for NO change
- You chose to support it through your efforts of thinking, planning, ruminating, etc.
- You chose to let your brain support it with your consent to habitual, unchecked thought.

Choice for change
- You choose to change you habitual thought patterns and to practice a different relationship to the content.

Body:

Choose to acknowledge that your pelvic pain may have resulted from faulty storage and retrieval.

PS53 Other Activities Of Your Life

Mental:

Different functional areas of your brain are involved in the maintenance of the stories of your life. The functional areas communicate with each other.

Choose other activities that will require interaction between the different functional areas of your brain.

Body:

Remember to take advantage of novel activities during your day. These are opportunities to identify areas of practice.

PS54 Allocation Process

Mental:

Training your attentional skills and using your attentional skills affects the process of allocating resources, processes that are **not within your ability to observe**.

This change in allocation process is very important. Allocation in support of your chosen values is a very skillful use of your scarce resources.

It is desirable to train your brain to handle this allocation decision **without displaying the process in your field of awareness.**

Acknowledge that your desired changes in allocation are facilitated when you **choose to work with your thought and emotion content throughout your day when presented with an opportunity**.

Body:

Feature the sense of being a witness of the sensations in your pelvis.

PS55 Training

Mental:

Attentional resources are trained through the sitting practices and through the practice with content throughout your day.

Body:

Sometime during the day choose to **practice a remembrance** of your pelvic pain. Tune into the area that you think the pain comes from and see if you can remember what it felt like – as many characteristics of the pain experience as you can recall. See if you can find where it was located in your body and remember what it felt like – intensity, duration, other qualities. At that moment, consider if you can remember related feelings or sensations in other parts of your body (head, face, neck, shoulders, abdomen, limbs).

PS56 Being An Observer

Mental:

A different relationship to your thoughts, that of being an "observer", is learned through the sitting practices and through the practice with content throughout your day.

Body:

It can be very useful to make frequent use of the full body scan.

"Take an inventory" of your body. With this inventory **feature felt sensations**. Briefly note the quality, intensity or other characteristics of the felt sensation.

Begin at your feet and move up your body with your examination – feet, ankle, calf, knee, thigh, hips, buttocks, pelvic area, abdomen, spine, chest, back, shoulders, upper arm, lower arm, hand, neck, face and head.

PS57 Choices

Mental:

You are the only one that can observe the habits of your own brain.

You have a choice to make when you observe habitual thought content that does not serve your interest.

- Choose to become involved.
- Choose to NOT become involved, to allow the habitual content to be maintained.

Body:

Chronic pain is not the same as acute pain. Chronic pain may begin with tissue damage, but can be perpetuated by other factors long after a reasonable time has passed for healing. It becomes a habit.

Choose to become involved. Choose to feature purposeful actions to provide information for a solution.

PS58 Involved

Mental:

If you choose to become involved in the untangling of this content that does not serve your interest, the initial two-part response remains:

- **Acknowledge** with simple comments: There is a thought. This is what the brain does. My brain contributes random thoughts. What it contributes may not be useful.
- **Redirect**: Choose to bring your attention back to a focus of your choice.

Body:

Choose to practice **specifically focusing on felt senses** using full body scan featuring the body parts that you have identified as needing more attention. Choose to focus on sensations.

PS59 Other Work With Content

Mental:

If you choose to become involved in the untangling of this content that does not serve your interest, additional cognitive work with the content is within your interest.

There are many options for externally focused **conscious, cognitive work** with your content including self-help, group work in a community of your choice, and *professional help*.

Body:

Remember to take advantage of novel activities during your day. These are opportunities to identify areas of practice.

PS60 As Best You Can

Mental:

"As best you can."

Body:

Committing to becoming involved (with intention to evaluate and identify action plans to affect posture, position, and changes in position) instigates different cognitive processes that support goal achievement.

Bibliographic Information
(in order of occurrence)

Urologic Chronic Pelvic Pain Syndrome (UCPPS) Research (R01). National Institutes of Health Web site. http://grants.nih.gov/grants/guide/rfa-files/RFA-DK-12-025.html. Published November 30, 2012. Accessed September 1, 2013.

Sabate E. 2003. *Adherence to Long-Term Therapies: Evidence for Action.* Geneva: World Health Organ.

Jin J, Sklar GE, Min Sen Oh V, Chuen Li S. Factors affecting therapeutic compliance: A review from the patient's perspective. Ther Clin Risk Manag. 2008; 4(1): 269–286.

Eamon Fulcher. *Cognitive Psychology.* Exeter, UK: Learning Matters Ltd; 2003.

Posner MI, Peterson SE. The attention system of the human brain. Annu Rev Neurosci. 1990; 13: 25–42.

Lutz A, Slagter HA, Dunne J, Davidson RJ. Attention regulation and monitoring in meditation. Trends Cogn. Sci. 2008; 12: 163–169.

The Oxford Dictionary of Sports Science & Medicine. 3rd ed. New York, NY: Oxford University Press; 2007.

McCallum CW. "Attention." *Encyclopaedia Britannica.* 2007. *Britannica Online.* Web. 29 Sept. 2013.

Dickens C. *A Christmas Carol. In Prose. Being a Ghost Story of Christmas.* London: Chapman and Hall; 1843.

Hu JC, Link CL, McNaughton-Collins M, Barry MJ, McKinlay JB. The association of abuse and symptoms suggestive of chronic prostatitis/chronic pelvic pain syndrome: results from the Boston Area Community Health survey. J Gen Intern Med. 2007; 22(11): 1532–7.

Fedorak C, Ashworth N, Marshall J, Paull H. Reliability of the visual assessment of cervical and lumbar lordosis: how good are we? Spine. 2003; 28(16): 1857-9.

Jerath R, Edry JW, Barnes VA, Jerath V. Physiology of long pranayamic breathing: neural respiratory elements may provide a mechanism that explains how slow deep breathing shifts the autonomic nervous system. Med Hypotheses. 2006; 67(3): 566–71.

Acknowledgment of Inspiration

Thoughts are our inner senses.
John O'Donohue, *Anam Cara*, p. 17.

Richard Davidson
Rex Jung
Zindel V. Segal, J. Mark G. Williams, John D. Teasdale
Andrew Newberg
Tania Singer
Roy F. Baumeister
Willoughby Britton
Krista Tippet
Paul Gilbert
Cathy Kerr
Leon Chaitow
J. C. Nickel
D. A. Tripp
Ted Robinson
Tim Parks

www.pelvicpain-cpps.com/inspiration

Author's Bio

Lea Wilson is new to nonfiction publishing. Her career has included diverse "nonfiction" writing - from patient education materials to policy and procedure manuals. She was writing a book about *teaching meditation without the dharma in the Bible belt* when she was side-tracked by her husband's chronic pelvic pain. She has degrees in Sociology and Clinical Nutrition and is a Certified Public Accountant. You can contact her at leawilson1342@yahoo.com or the website www.pelvicpain-cpps.com.